Introduction

As the author of this book, I want to begin by expressing my deep gratitude for your interest in this important topic.

Gout, a condition that affects millions of people around the world, has been a significant part of my personal journey. It is my hope that the knowledge and insights shared within these pages will prove invaluable to you or your loved ones as you navigate the challenges of gout.

The Inspiration behind Writing this Book

My Brother-in-law, Lenny's experiences with gout served as the catalyst for this book. Like many of you, he had to confront the agonizing pain and frustration that comes with a Gout and Kidney stones diagnosis. The relentless joint pain, the sudden flare-ups in his feet, the recurrence of new kidney stones and the limitations it imposed on his life were experiences I wouldn't wish upon anyone.

But with his challenging moments, drove me to do some research on what causes gout, and I found inspiration. I discovered the healing philosophies of Dr. Sebi and his emphasis on the power of nature and herbalistic remedies. Dr. Sebi's work resonated with me on a profound level, offering a glimmer of hope and the promise of relief for my Brother-in-Law. The journey to understand and apply his teachings became a transformative experience that I felt compelled to share with others facing the same struggle.

What Readers Can Expect to Learn and Achieve

This book is not just a compilation of information; it is a roadmap to empowerment and healing. Here's what you can expect to gain from its pages:

- **Understanding**: We'll start by unraveling the complexity of gout—what it is, why it happens, and why its prevalence continues to rise in the modern world. This understanding is crucial in paving the way for effective solutions.

- **Dr. Sebi's Wisdom**: Dr. Sebi's herbalistic philosophy is at the core of this guide. You'll dive deep into his principles, exploring the significance of an alkaline diet and the healing potential of specific herbs. These principles form the foundation for a holistic approach to gout relief.

- **Practical Guidance**: This book offers practical advice on implementing Dr. Sebi's approach in your daily life. You'll find meal plans, recipes, smoothies and step-by-step instructions on preparing and using herbal remedies. We'll also explore the importance of detoxification, hydration, and lifestyle modifications.

- **Challenges and Solutions**: Gout management is not without its obstacles. We'll address common challenges and provide strategies for overcoming them. Whether it's dealing with flare-ups or staying motivated, you'll find guidance to help you stay the course.

- **A Glimpse into the Future**: In the final chapters, we'll explore the evolving landscape of gout treatment in 2023. We'll discuss how modern healthcare is integrating herbalistic wisdom and the hope for a gout-free future.

It is my sincerest hope that this book becomes a valuable resource on your journey to eliminate gout and regain your health and vitality. Remember that you are not alone in this endeavor. Together, we will explore the holistic path to gout relief, armed with the wisdom of Dr. Sebi and the shared experiences of those who have walked this road before you.

As we embark on this enlightening and transformative journey, I invite you to approach these pages with an open heart and a willingness to explore the possibilities of natural healing. Let this book be your guide and companion on the path to a gout-free and vibrant life.

With warm regards,

Milo S. Sullivan

Contents

<u>**Chapter 1: Understanding Gout**</u>

Gout Unveiled: Understanding the Painful Reality

Gout, the often excruciatingly painful condition caused by the buildup of uric acid crystals in the joints, is on the rise in the modern world. In the year 2023, its prevalence has reached alarming levels, affecting millions of people worldwide. It's not just a disease of the past; it's a pressing concern for the present and future.

The Prevalence of Gout in Modern Society

To comprehend the gravity of the gout problem in 2023, we must first grasp its prevalence. In the United States alone, the number of gout cases has steadily increased over the years, making it one of the most common forms of arthritis. Affecting both men and women, gout doesn't discriminate based on gender or age. It can strike anyone, at any time, causing severe joint pain, inflammation, and a diminished quality of life.

The Urgent Need for Natural Solutions

Conventional treatments for gout often include medications like nonsteroidal anti-inflammatory drugs (NSAIDs) and urate-lowering drugs, which aim to manage symptoms and reduce uric acid levels. While these pharmaceutical interventions can provide temporary relief, they often come with side effects and limitations.

This is where the urgent need for natural solutions becomes apparent. Many individuals are seeking alternative methods to not only alleviate their gout symptoms but to eliminate the root causes of this debilitating condition. It is in this search for holistic, effective solutions that the herbalistic philosophies of Dr. Sebi shine.

Dr. Sebi's Legacy: A Trailblazer in Herbalistic Healing

Before delving into Dr. Sebi's approach to gout, it's essential to understand the man behind the philosophy.

Dr. Sebi, whose real name was Alfredo Darrington Bowman, was a Honduran herbalist and healer who dedicated his life to promoting natural healing methods. His journey began when he was diagnosed with asthma, diabetes, and obesity. Frustrated with conventional medicine's inability to provide a cure, he embarked on a quest to discover the healing power of nature. Through extensive research and experimentation, he developed a unique herbalistic approach that emphasized the importance of an alkaline diet and the use of specific herbs to address various health conditions, including gout.

How Dr. Sebi's Philosophy Can Transform Gout Management

Dr. Sebi's herbalistic philosophies have the potential to revolutionize the way we perceive and manage gout. By focusing on the principles of an alkaline diet and the use of specific herbs, his approach aims not only to alleviate gout symptoms but to address the underlying causes, ultimately leading to the elimination of this painful condition.

In the chapters that follow, we will delve deeper into his teachings, exploring the components of his alkaline diet, the power of herbal remedies, and the holistic approach to gout prevention and healing. By the end of this book, you will have a comprehensive understanding of how to apply Dr. Sebi's herbalistic wisdom to your own journey toward gout elimination.

As we embark on this exploration of gout relief through Dr. Sebi's herbalistic lens, keep in mind that you are not alone in your quest for a gout-free life. Many have walked this path before you, and their stories of success and transformation serve as beacons of hope. In the chapters that follow, we will uncover the tools and knowledge you need to take control of your gout and embark on a journey toward lasting relief and well-being.

Chapter 2: The Gout Challenge

The Growing Epidemic: Gout's Rise in the 21st Century

To comprehend the gravity of the gout problem in 2023, we must first grasp its prevalence. In the United States alone, the number of gout cases has steadily increased over the years, making it one of the most common forms of arthritis. Affecting both men and women, gout doesn't discriminate based on gender or age. It can strike anyone, at any time, causing severe joint pain, inflammation, and a diminished quality of life.

The 21st century has witnessed a striking rise in the occurrence of gout. This increase can be attributed to various factors, including changes in diet, lifestyle, and an aging population. While gout has been a recognized medical condition for centuries, its resurgence in recent years has prompted a reevaluation of how we approach its prevention and management.

Exploring Gout's Prevalence and Impact

Gout, often characterized by sudden and excruciatingly painful attacks, occurs when uric acid crystals accumulate in the joints. These crystals trigger inflammation, leading to intense pain and swelling, most commonly affecting the big toe but also other joints such as the ankles, knees, and wrists.

Statistics reveal a sobering reality: gout is on the rise. In the United States, it is estimated that over eight million adults suffer from gout, a number that has increased substantially in the past decade. Gout is not limited to the U.S.; it is a global health concern. Countries worldwide are grappling with a growing number of gout cases, impacting individuals, families, and healthcare systems.

The Limitations of Conventional Gout Treatments

Conventional treatments for gout often rely on medications aimed at managing symptoms and reducing uric acid levels. These approaches include nonsteroidal anti-inflammatory drugs (NSAIDs) to alleviate pain during acute attacks and urate-lowering drugs like Aloprim & Zyloprim (also known as **Allopurinol**) to treat gout and kidney stones or Uloric (also known as **Febuxostat**) to control uric acid production.

Common side effects of **Allopurinol** may include:

1. **Skin Rash:** This is one of the most common side effects. It can range from mild to severe. If you experience a rash while taking Allopurinol, it's crucial to contact your healthcare provider.

2. **Digestive Issues:** Some people may experience gastrointestinal symptoms like nausea, vomiting, or diarrhea.

3. **Headache:** Headaches can occur in some individuals as a side effect.

4. **Elevated Liver Enzymes:** May lead to increased levels of liver enzymes in some individuals, which would be detected through blood tests.

5. **Kidney Problems:** In rare cases, may affect kidney function, leading to kidney problems.

6. **Hypersensitivity Reactions:** Severe allergic reactions, though rare, can occur. Symptoms may include fever, swollen lymph nodes, skin rash, and more.

Common side effects of **<u>Febuxostat</u>** may include:

1. **Nausea:** Some individuals may experience mild to moderate nausea.

2. **Joint Pain:** Joint pain, which can mimic gout symptoms, is a possible side effect.

3. **Rash:** Skin rash is another potential side effect.

4. **Liver Enzyme Elevation:** An increase in liver enzymes, which can be detected through blood tests.

5. **Digestive Issues:** Gastrointestinal symptoms such as diarrhea or stomach pain can occur.

6. **Headache:** Some individuals may experience headaches.

7. **Allergic Reactions:** While rare, severe allergic reactions can occur. Symptoms may include hives, difficulty breathing, swelling of the face or throat, and more.

It's important to take **Allopurinol** or **Febuxostat** as prescribed by your healthcare provider and to promptly report any side effects or unusual symptoms to them. Your healthcare provider will evaluate whether the benefits of the medication outweigh the potential risks in your specific situation.

While these pharmaceutical interventions have their merits, they also have their shortcomings. NSAIDs may provide temporary relief, but they do not address the root causes of gout. Furthermore, they can lead to gastrointestinal issues and other side effects when used extensively.

Urate-lowering drugs, on the other hand, aim to reduce uric acid levels in the body, which can help prevent future gout attacks. However, these drugs may take time to show their effects and are not without potential side effects such as skin rashes and liver problems. Additionally, they may not be suitable for everyone.

It is in recognizing the limitations of conventional gout treatments that many individuals are seeking alternative, natural approaches to gout management. They yearn for solutions that not only provide relief from symptoms but also address the root causes of gout, paving the way for lasting freedom from this painful condition.

Chapter 3: Dr. Sebi's Healing Principles

The Foundation of Healing: An Alkaline Diet

Understanding the Alkaline Food List

To embark on our journey into Dr. Sebi's herbalistic approach to gout, we must first delve into the cornerstone of his healing philosophy—the alkaline diet. He believed that maintaining an alkaline state in the body is essential for overall health and well-being, and this belief forms the basis of his approach to gout relief.

An alkaline diet is one that emphasizes foods that have an alkalizing effect on the body. The opposite of an alkaline diet is an acidic one, which includes foods that create an acidic environment within the body. He advocated for consuming predominantly alkaline foods to restore balance and promote healing.

To get a clear understanding of what constitutes an alkaline diet, it's helpful to examine the alkaline food list. This list categorizes foods into alkaline, neutral, and acidic groups based on their impact on the body's pH levels.

High-Alkaline Foods for Gout Relief

Dr. Sebi's alkaline food list includes a wide variety of fruits, vegetables, nuts, seeds, and grains that are known for their alkalizing properties. These foods are not only nutrient-dense but also play a vital role in maintaining the body's alkaline balance.

Some examples of high-alkaline foods recommended by Dr. Sebi include leafy greens like kale and spinach, fruits such as avocados and lemons, nuts like almonds and walnuts, and whole grains like quinoa and spelt. These foods are rich in essential vitamins, minerals, and antioxidants, making them an integral part of a gout-preventive diet.

Meal Planning and Delicious Recipes

Transitioning to an alkaline diet can be a rewarding but sometimes challenging journey. To help you make this shift, we'll explore practical strategies for meal planning and preparation. You'll discover how to create balanced and delicious meals that align with Dr. Sebi's alkaline principles.

Whether you're new to the concept of an alkaline diet or looking to enhance your existing knowledge, the recipes and meal ideas presented in this chapter will provide you with inspiration and guidance. From vibrant salads to hearty grain bowls and satisfying smoothies, you'll have a wealth of options to choose from, all designed to support your gout relief journey.

The Alkaline Diet in Action: Success Stories

Understanding the alkaline diet is one thing, but witnessing its impact on real people's lives is another. In this chapter, we'll explore the stories of individuals who have embraced Dr. Sebi's alkaline principles and experienced remarkable transformations in their gout management.

These success stories serve as compelling evidence of the healing potential of an alkaline diet. You'll find inspiration in the journeys of those who have not only alleviated their gout symptoms but also improved their overall health and vitality through the power of alkaline nutrition.

As we dive deeper into Dr. Sebi's alkaline diet and its role in gout relief, keep in mind that this dietary approach is not a one-size-fits-all solution. It is a flexible framework that can be tailored to your individual preferences and needs. Whether you're looking to prevent gout or seeking relief from its symptoms, the alkaline diet offers a natural and holistic path toward healing.

In the chapters ahead, we'll continue to explore Dr. Sebi's healing principles, delving into the specifics of his herbal remedies and how they can complement your journey to eliminate gout naturally.

Chapter 4: Gout Unveiled

Unmasking the Root Causes of Gout

To effectively address any health condition, including gout, it's essential to understand its root causes. In this chapter, we'll delve deep into the factors that contribute to the development of gout and how they align with Dr. Sebi's herbalistic philosophy.

The Complex Interplay of Genetics and Lifestyle

Gout is not solely the result of one factor but rather a complex interplay of genetic predisposition and lifestyle choices. While genetics can play a role in an individual's susceptibility to gout, lifestyle factors often serve as the triggers that lead to gout attacks.

Certain genetic factors can make some people more prone to producing higher levels of uric acid, a key contributor to gout. However, genetics alone do not guarantee the development of gout. Lifestyle choices, particularly dietary habits and levels of physical activity, can significantly influence whether gout manifests.

The Role of Diet in Gout Development

Dietary choices, particularly the consumption of purine-rich foods, are major contributors to gout development. Purines are natural compounds found in various foods and are broken down into uric acid in the body. When uric acid levels become too high, crystals can form and accumulate in the joints, leading to gout attacks.

Foods high in purines include red meat, organ meats (such as liver and kidney), certain seafood (like shellfish and anchovies), and alcoholic beverages. These items are commonly associated with gout flare-ups.

How Dr. Sebi's Approach Addresses Gout's Underlying Causes

Dr. Sebi's herbalistic approach to gout aligns with the understanding that gout is not just a symptom to be managed but a condition to be addressed at its source. His teachings emphasize that the body has an innate ability to heal itself when provided with the right nutrients and conditions.

By adopting an alkaline diet, you create an environment in which uric acid crystals are less likely to form and trigger gout attacks. Alkaline foods help neutralize excess acidity in the body, reducing the risk of crystal formation.

Additionally, Dr. Sebi's recommended herbs play a pivotal role in gout prevention and relief. Certain herbs possess properties that can assist the body in breaking down and eliminating uric acid more effectively. They also support overall kidney function, which is vital for excreting uric acid from the body.

As we journey further into this book, we will explore the specific herbs and herbal remedies that he advocated for gout relief. We'll uncover the science behind their effectiveness and provide practical guidance on how to incorporate them into your daily routine.

Remember, understanding the root causes of gout is the first step toward effective and lasting relief. With Dr. Sebi's herbalistic wisdom as our guide, we'll continue on the path toward gout elimination in the chapters that follow.

Chapter 5: Dr. Sebi's Alkaline Diet

A Detailed Examination of the Alkaline Food List

Understanding the Alkaline Food List is fundamental to adopting Dr. Sebi's herbalistic approach to gout relief. In this chapter, we will delve deeper into the specifics of the alkaline diet, exploring the foods you should prioritize and those you should limit or avoid.

High-Alkaline Foods for Gout Relief

Dr. Sebi's alkaline food list categorizes foods into three primary groups: alkaline, neutral, and acidic. Alkaline foods are the foundation of this dietary approach, and they are known for their ability to maintain or restore the body's alkaline balance.

Here are some examples of high-alkaline foods that Dr. Sebi recommended for gout relief:

1. **Leafy Greens**: Kale, spinach, collard greens, and Swiss chard are excellent choices. They are rich in essential nutrients and have a strong alkalizing effect on the body.

2. **Fruits**: Avocados, lemons, limes, and grapes are alkaline fruits that can be enjoyed to support your gout-preventive diet.

3. **Nuts and Seeds**: Almonds, walnuts, and flaxseeds are among the nuts and seeds that align with the alkaline principles.

4. **Whole Grains**: Quinoa, spelt, and amaranth are whole grains that are considered alkaline. They provide valuable fiber and nutrients.

5. **Herbal Teas**: Certain herbal teas, such as chamomile and peppermint, can be included in your alkaline diet plan.

6. **Spices and Seasonings**: Dr. Sebi advocated for the use of natural herbs and seasonings like basil, thyme, and cayenne pepper to add flavor to your meals while staying alkaline.

These high-alkaline foods not only support gout relief but also contribute to overall health and vitality. They are packed with vitamins, minerals, antioxidants, and other essential nutrients that your body craves.

Meal Planning and Delicious Recipes

Transitioning to an alkaline diet doesn't mean sacrificing flavor or variety in your meals. In fact, there are numerous delicious and satisfying recipes that align with Dr. Sebi's principles.

From refreshing salads with vibrant greens and a medley of colorful vegetables to hearty grain bowls bursting with flavor, you'll discover a world of culinary possibilities that support your gout prevention and relief efforts.

As you explore these recipes and meal ideas, keep in mind that the alkaline diet is flexible and can be tailored to your preferences. Whether you're a fan of plant-based cuisine or looking to incorporate alkaline principles into your existing dietary habits, there's room for creativity and adaptation.

By the end of this chapter, you'll have a deeper understanding of how to build nourishing, alkaline meals that not only taste great but also contribute to your journey toward gout elimination. The alkaline diet is not a temporary solution but a sustainable way of eating that can transform your health and well-being.

<u>**Chapter 6: Herbal Allies in Gout Elimination**</u>

Dr. Sebi's Arsenal of Herbal Remedies

In this chapter, we will explore Dr. Sebi's recommended herbs and how they play a pivotal role in gout prevention and relief. He firmly believed in the healing power of nature, and his herbalistic approach to health offers valuable insights into harnessing the potential of herbs for gout elimination.

An In-Depth Look at Key Gout-Fighting Herbs

Dr. Sebi identified several herbs that he believed to be particularly effective in addressing the underlying causes of gout and providing relief from its symptoms. These herbs are carefully selected for their ability to support the body's natural healing processes.

Some of the key herbs recommended by Dr. Sebi for gout relief include:

1. **Burdock Root**: Burdock root is known for its anti-inflammatory properties and its potential to aid in the elimination of toxins from the body. It can be particularly beneficial in reducing gout-related inflammation. https://amzn.to/46a9nTj

2. **Nettle**: Nettle is a natural diuretic that may help the body flush excess uric acid, a contributing factor to gout attacks. It also contains anti-inflammatory compounds that can provide relief from joint pain. https://amzn.to/3rc6NNF

3. **Dandelion**: Dandelion is another diuretic herb that supports kidney function. Proper kidney function is essential for the excretion of uric acid, making dandelion a valuable ally in gout prevention. https://amzn.to/46aKMh3

4. **Devil's Claw**: Devil's claw is renowned for its anti-inflammatory properties. It may help reduce pain and inflammation associated with gout attacks, improving overall comfort. https://amzn.to/3PiWI9L

5. **Bromide Plus Powder**: Dr. Sebi's Bromide Plus Powder is a proprietary blend of herbs designed to support various aspects of health, including gout relief. It contains sea moss, Bladderwrack, and other ingredients that align with the alkaline diet and herbal philosophy. www.drsebiscellfood.com

These herbs are just a few examples of the many natural remedies that Dr. Sebi recommended for gout management. They can be used individually or combined in herbal preparations to create potent remedies that address gout's root causes and provide relief from its symptoms. To purchase these herbs...Click on the link for each herb.

Creating and Administering Herbal Remedies

While it's possible to find commercial herbal products that contain Dr. Sebi's recommended herbs, many individuals choose to prepare their herbal remedies at home. This allows for customization and ensures the use of high-quality ingredients.

In this chapter, we will provide step-by-step guidance on how to create and administer herbal remedies for gout relief. You'll learn about various preparation methods, including teas, tinctures, and capsules, and how to determine the right dosage for your specific needs.

By the end of this chapter, you'll have a comprehensive understanding of his herbalistic approach to gout elimination and the practical knowledge needed to incorporate these herbal remedies into your daily routine.

As we continue our journey through this book, we'll explore the importance of detoxification, hydration, and lifestyle modifications in gout management, complementing the herbal wisdom of Dr. Sebi.

Chapter 7: Detoxification and Gout

The Vital Role of Detoxification in Gout Management

Detoxification is a crucial aspect of Dr. Sebi's herbalistic approach to gout management. In this chapter, we'll explore why detoxification is essential, how toxins contribute to gout flare-ups, and Dr. Sebi's detox protocols and their benefits.

How Toxins Contribute to Gout Flare-Ups

The human body is exposed to a wide range of toxins from various sources, including the environment, food, and lifestyle choices. Over time, the accumulation of these toxins can overwhelm the body's natural detoxification systems, leading to a buildup of waste and metabolic byproducts.

For individuals with gout, this accumulation of toxins can be particularly problematic. Toxins can contribute to inflammation and oxidative stress in the body, both of which are known triggers for gout attacks. Additionally, toxins can burden the kidneys, which play a crucial role in excreting uric acid. When the kidneys are compromised due to toxin overload, uric acid levels can rise, increasing the risk of gout.

Dr. Sebi's Detox Protocols and Their Benefits

Dr. Sebi advocated for regular detoxification as a means to eliminate toxins from the body and support overall health. His detox protocols involve a combination of fasting, herbal remedies, and dietary adjustments.

Some of the key benefits of detoxification in gout management include:

1. **Reduced Inflammation**: Detoxification can help reduce inflammation in the body, which is a common trigger for gout attacks.

2. **Improved Kidney Function**: By relieving the kidneys of the burden of toxins, detoxification supports their ability to excrete uric acid efficiently.

3. **Enhanced Cellular Health**: Detoxification at the cellular level promotes optimal function and may reduce the risk of uric acid crystal formation.

4. **Balanced pH Levels**: Detoxification can contribute to maintaining the body's pH balance, making it less conducive to uric acid crystal formation.

In this chapter, we'll delve into the practical aspects of detoxification, including different detox methods you can explore and how to incorporate them into your gout management plan. Whether you choose to embark on a full detox program or make gradual lifestyle changes to support ongoing detoxification, you'll discover valuable insights and strategies.

Detox Success Stories: Stories of Triumph over Gout

To inspire and motivate you on your detox journey, we'll also share success stories of individuals who have experienced remarkable transformations through detoxification. These real-life accounts highlight the profound impact that detox can have on gout relief and overall well-being. By the end of this chapter, you'll have a comprehensive understanding of the importance of detoxification in gout management and the practical steps you can take to incorporate detox protocols into your holistic approach to gout elimination.

As we continue our exploration, we'll delve into the significance of hydration for gout prevention and relief, providing you with practical tips and techniques to ensure you stay adequately hydrated

<u>**Chapter 8: Hydration and Gout Relief**</u>

The Crucial Role of Hydration in Gout Management

Proper hydration is a fundamental aspect of gout relief and prevention, and Dr. Sebi emphasized its significance in his herbalistic approach. In this chapter, we'll explore why staying hydrated is essential for gout management and provide practical guidance on how to ensure you're getting enough fluids.

Why Hydration Matters in Gout Relief

Water is often referred to as the "universal solvent" because of its ability to dissolve a wide range of substances, including uric acid crystals. When you're well-hydrated, your body can more effectively flush out excess uric acid, reducing the risk of crystal formation in the joints.

Inadequate hydration, on the other hand, can lead to uric acid buildup, making gout attacks more likely and more painful. Dehydration can also contribute to joint stiffness and discomfort.

Dr. Sebi's Approach to Hydration

Dr. Sebi recommended a specific approach to hydration that aligns with his herbalistic philosophy. While water is undoubtedly a primary source of hydration, he also emphasized the importance of incorporating natural, alkaline-rich beverages into your daily routine.

Some of the key elements of Dr. Sebi's hydration approach include:

1. **Alkaline Water**: Drinking alkaline water, which has a higher pH level than regular tap water, can help maintain the body's alkaline balance. Alkaline water is believed to be more effective in neutralizing excess acidity in the body.

2. **Herbal Teas**: Certain herbal teas, such as chamomile and peppermint, can contribute to hydration while providing additional health benefits. These teas are not only soothing but also align with Dr. Sebi's alkaline principles.

3. **Fresh Fruit Juices**: Dr. Sebi encouraged the consumption of fresh fruit juices, particularly those made from alkaline fruits like lemons and limes. These juices are not only hydrating but also provide essential vitamins and minerals.

4. **Hydrating Foods**: Many fruits and vegetables have high water content and can contribute to your daily hydration needs. Incorporating these foods into your diet is a practical way to stay hydrated.

Practical Hydration Tips and Strategies

In this chapter, we'll provide practical tips and strategies to ensure you stay adequately hydrated on your journey to gout relief. You'll discover how to establish a hydration routine that works for you, how to monitor your hydration levels, and how to make mindful beverage choices that align with Dr. Sebi's principles.

Remember that hydration is not just about the quantity of fluids you consume but also the quality. By incorporating alkaline-rich beverages and hydrating foods into your diet, you'll support your body's natural detoxification processes and reduce the risk of gout attacks.

As we progress through the remaining chapters of this book, we'll delve into lifestyle modifications and holistic strategies that complement Dr. Sebi's herbalistic wisdom, all aimed at helping you achieve gout elimination in 2023 and beyond.

Creating a Gout-Friendly Lifestyle

In this chapter, we'll explore the importance of lifestyle modifications in your journey to eliminate gout naturally. Dr. Sebi's herbalistic approach goes beyond diet and herbs—it encompasses a holistic way of living that promotes overall health and well-being.

Exercise and Gout

Physical activity plays a crucial role in gout management. Regular exercise helps maintain a healthy weight, which is essential for reducing the risk of gout attacks. It also improves joint flexibility and can alleviate gout-related stiffness and discomfort.

However, it's essential to approach exercise with caution, especially during gout flare-ups. In this chapter, we'll provide guidance on suitable exercise routines for gout relief and strategies to stay active while minimizing the risk of exacerbating symptoms.

Stress Management

Stress is a known trigger for gout attacks. When you're stressed, your body releases hormones that can increase inflammation and uric acid levels. Learning effective stress management techniques is crucial for gout prevention.

In this chapter, we'll explore mindfulness practices, relaxation techniques, and lifestyle adjustments that can help you reduce stress and its impact on gout. These strategies will not only benefit your gout management but also enhance your overall quality of life.

Quality Sleep

Getting adequate and restful sleep is vital for your body's natural healing processes Poor sleep patterns can contribute to inflammation and may increase the likelihood of gout attacks. We'll discuss sleep hygiene tips and strategies to help you improve the quality and duration of your sleep.

Alcohol and Gout

Alcohol consumption is a well-known risk factor for gout. Certain alcoholic beverages, such as beer and spirits, are high in purines and can lead to increased uric acid levels. We'll explore the impact of alcohol on gout and provide guidance on making mindful choices when it comes to drinking.

Gout-Friendly Supplements

While Dr. Sebi's approach primarily focuses on herbal remedies and whole foods, some supplements may complement your gout management plan. In this chapter, we'll discuss specific supplements that align with Dr. Sebi's principles and may offer additional support in your journey to gout relief.

By the end of this chapter, you'll have a comprehensive understanding of the lifestyle modifications that can enhance your gout management efforts. These modifications are not isolated strategies but interconnected components of a holistic approach to gout elimination.

As we approach the conclusion of this book, we'll look ahead to the evolving landscape of gout treatment in 2023, exploring how modern healthcare is integrating herbalistic wisdom and offering hope for a gout-free future.

<u>**Chapter 10: The Future of Gout Treatment in 2023 and Beyond**</u>

A Gout-Free Future

In this final chapter, we'll look ahead to the evolving landscape of gout treatment in 2023 and beyond. The integration of herbalistic wisdom and modern healthcare offers hope for a future where gout can be effectively prevented and managed.

The Bridging of Traditions: Herbalistic Wisdom and Modern Medicine

The herbalistic philosophy of Dr. Sebi, with its emphasis on natural remedies and holistic healing, has gained recognition and acceptance within the realm of modern medicine. As a result, we are witnessing a convergence of traditional wisdom and scientific innovation in the treatment of gout.

Medical researchers and healthcare professionals are increasingly exploring the potential of herbal remedies, dietary adjustments, and lifestyle modifications in gout management. This collaborative approach acknowledges that gout is not just a symptom to be managed but a condition that can be addressed at its source.

The Promise of Personalized Medicine

One of the exciting developments in gout treatment is the emergence of personalized medicine. This approach recognizes that each individual's experience with gout is unique, and treatments should be tailored to their specific needs and genetic makeup.

Advancements in genetic testing and research allow healthcare providers to identify genetic factors that may contribute to gout susceptibility. This information can inform personalized treatment plans that address the root causes of gout in a way that is uniquely suited to the individual.

The Role of Dietary Science

Dietary science continues to play a pivotal role in gout management. Researchers are delving into the relationship between diet, gut health, and gout development. This knowledge is leading to more precise dietary recommendations and interventions that target the underlying causes of gout.

Holistic Healthcare

The holistic approach to healthcare is gaining momentum. This approach recognizes that the body is an interconnected system, and addressing one aspect of health can have ripple effects throughout the entire body. As we've explored in this book, holistic strategies, including detoxification, hydration, and stress management, are crucial components of gout relief.

The Empowered Gout Warrior

In this final chapter, we want to emphasize the importance of empowerment. By arming yourself with knowledge about gout, herbalistic wisdom, and the evolving landscape of gout treatment, you become an empowered gout warrior.

Gout may have once seemed like an insurmountable challenge, but with the right information and resources, you have the ability to take control of your health and work towards gout elimination. Your journey may involve a combination of herbal remedies, dietary adjustments, lifestyle modifications, and personalized medical interventions. The future of gout treatment is brighter than ever, and you are at the forefront of this exciting evolution.

<u>Closing Thoughts</u>

As we conclude this book, we want to express our gratitude for accompanying us on this journey through the world of gout and herbalistic wisdom. Gout may have posed challenges in the past, but armed with the knowledge and a holistic approach, you have the potential to achieve a gout-free future in 2023 and beyond.

Remember that your health is your most valuable asset, and investing in it is a decision you won't regret. Whether you choose to embrace Dr. Sebi's herbalistic philosophy or explore modern healthcare innovations, the path to gout relief and elimination is within your reach.

Thank you for entrusting us with this part of your journey. Let your future be filled with vibrant health, vitality, and the freedom to live your life to the fullest.

<u>**Appendix: Resources and References**</u>

In your journey to eliminate gout naturally and embrace Dr. Sebi's herbalistic wisdom, it's essential to have access to valuable resources and references. This appendix provides a curated list of sources, books, websites, and organizations that can further support your quest for gout relief and holistic well-being. *Click the link to purchase these books.*

Books and Publications

1. *Dr. Sebi's Alkaline and Anti-Inflammatory Diet for Beginners* by **Serena Brown** - How to Naturally Reduce Inflammation and Boost Immunity for Life-Long Health | Alkaline Diet | and includes a 28 day Detox Plan... & More! (https://amzn.to/45G8P7W)

2. *The Healing Gout Cookbook: Anti-Inflammatory Recipes to Lower Uric Acid Levels and Reduce Flares* by **Lisa Cicciarello Andrews** - The Healing Gout Cookbook is your guide to a nourishing, anti-inflammatory diet full of fresh and flavorful foods with these 85 simple & satisfying recipes. (https://amzn.to/463U2n0)

3. *The 28-Day Gout Diet Plan: The Optimal Nutrition Guide to Manage Gout* by **Sophia Kamveris** - A gout-friendly diet plays a significant role in reducing painful flares for long-term treatment. (https://amzn.to/3ZawJWr)

4. *The China Study* by **Dr. T. Colin Campbell and Thomas M. Campbell II** - While not specific to gout, this book explores the health benefits of a plant-based diet and may inspire dietary changes aligned with Dr. Sebi's principles. (https://amzn.to/3sCJqx6)

Websites and Online Resources

1. **Dr. Sebi's Official Website** (www.drsebiscellfood.com) - This website provides information about Dr. Sebi's teachings, herbal products, and nutritional guidelines.

2. **The Gout & You Website** (www.goutandyou.com) - An informative resource on gout management, offering articles, recipes, and practical advice.

3. **National Institute of Arthritis and Musculoskeletal and Skin Diseases (NIAMS)** (www.niams.nih.gov) - A reputable source of information on various musculoskeletal conditions, including gout.

Herbal Remedies and Products

1. **Dr. Sebi's Cell Food** (www.drsebiscellfood.com) - The official source for Dr. Sebi's herbal products, including those recommended for gout relief.

2. **Mountain Rose Herbs** (www.mountainroseherbs.com) - A trusted supplier of high-quality herbs and herbal products for those interested in creating their herbal remedies.

Gout Support and Communities

1. **Gout and You Forum** (www.goutandyou.com/forum) - An online community where individuals affected by gout share their experiences and support one another.

2. **Arthritis Foundation** (www.arthritis.org) - An organization that offers resources, research, and support for individuals living with various forms of arthritis, including gout.

"These resources and references are meant to enhance the knowledge presented in this book and offer valuable aids in your quest to naturally alleviate gout. As you delve deeper into the realm of gout relief and holistic well-being, you may find these sources to be valuable for further understanding and assistance. (Please bear in mind that the availability and content of external websites and resources may evolve over time. It is advisable to verify the latest information and consult with healthcare professionals when making significant adjustments to your healthcare strategy.)"

Smoothie Drinks

(These kidney and gout-friendly smoothie recipes are not only delicious but are also aligned with Dr. Sebi's herbal alkaline diet principles. Enjoy these nourishing and kidney-friendly drinks as part of a balanced diet.)

1. Kidney Stone Crusher

- Ingredients:

    - 1 cup of watermelon chunks

    - 1/2 cucumber, peeled and chopped

    - 1/2 lemon, juiced

    - 1 tablespoon of fresh mint leaves

    - 1 teaspoon of chia seeds

    - 1 cup of coconut water

- Portion Measurements: 1 serving (approx. 16 oz)

- Nutritional Information (per serving):

    - Calories: 100

    - Carbohydrates: 24g

    - Fiber: 5g

    - Protein: 3g

    - Fat: 2g

- Prep Time: 5 minutes

- Instructions:

1. Combine watermelon chunks, cucumber, lemon juice, fresh mint leaves, chia seeds, and coconut water in a blender.

2. Blend until smooth and kidney stone-crushing!

3. Serve in a glass and toast to kidney health.

2. Gout Buster Blueberry Blast

- Ingredients:

  - 1 cup of blueberries

  - 1/2 banana

  - 1/2 cup of kale, stems removed

  - 1 tablespoon of flaxseed meal

  - 1/2 lime, juiced

  - 1 cup of coconut water

- Portion Measurements: 1 serving (approx. 16 oz)

- Nutritional Information (per serving):

  - Calories: 140

  - Carbohydrates: 30g

  - Fiber: 9g

  - Protein: 4g

  - Fat: 3g

- Prep Time: 5 minutes

- Instructions:

1. Blend blueberries, banana, kale, flaxseed meal, lime juice, and coconut water in a blender.

2. Blend until bursting with gout-fighting flavor.

3. Serve in a glass and savor the blueberry blast!

<u>**3. Stone Soothing Spinach Delight**</u>

- <u>Ingredients:</u>
    - <u>1 cup of spinach</u>
    - <u>1/2 cup of pineapple chunks</u>
    - <u>1/2 banana</u>
    - <u>1 tablespoon of hemp seeds</u>
    - <u>1/2 lemon, juiced</u>
    - <u>1 cup of coconut water</u>
- <u>Portion Measurements: 1 serving (approx. 16 oz.)</u>
- <u>Nutritional Information (per serving):</u>
    - <u>Calories: 190</u>
    - <u>Carbohydrates: 36g</u>
    - <u>Fiber: 6g</u>
    - <u>Protein: 6g</u>
    - <u>Fat: 4g</u>
- <u>Prep Time: 5 minutes</u>
- <u>Instructions:</u>

1. <u>Combine spinach, pineapple chunks, banana, hemp seeds, lemon juice, and coconut water in a blender.</u>

2. <u>Blend until soothing and delightful for your kidneys and gout.</u>

3. <u>Serve in a glass and relax with this stone-soothing blend!</u>

4. Cherry Kidney Cleanse

- Ingredients:

    - 1 cup of cherries (pitted)

    - 1/2 cup of cucumber, peeled and chopped

    - 1/2 lime, juiced

    - 1 tablespoon of chia seeds

    - 1 cup of coconut water

- Portion Measurements: 1 serving (approx. 16 oz.)

- Nutritional Information (per serving):

    - Calories: 140

    - Carbohydrates: 30g

    - Fiber: 6g

    - Protein: 3g

    - Fat: 3g

- Prep Time: 5 minutes

- Instructions:

1. Blend cherries, cucumber, lime juice, chia seeds, and coconut water in a blender.

2. Blend until kidney-cleansing and cherry-licious.

3. Serve in a glass and cleanse your kidneys with every sip!

5. Turmeric Twist Anti-Inflammatory Smoothie

- Ingredients:

    - 1/2 cup of pineapple chunks

    - 1/2 banana

    - 1/2 teaspoon of turmeric powder

    - 1/4 teaspoon of ginger powder

    - 1/2 lemon, juiced

    - 1 cup of coconut water

- Portion Measurements: 1 serving (approx. 16 oz.)

- Nutritional Information (per serving):

    - Calories: 130

    - Carbohydrates: 30g

    - Fiber: 5g

    - Protein: 2g

    - Fat: 1g

- Prep Time: 5 minutes

- Instructions:

1. Combine pineapple chunks, banana, turmeric powder, ginger powder, lemon juice, and coconut water in a blender.

2. Blend until anti-inflammatory and uniquely delicious.

3. Serve in a glass and enjoy the turmeric twist!

<u>**6. Lemonade Kidney Cleanser**</u>

- <u>Ingredients:</u>

    - <u>2 lemons, juiced</u>

    - <u>1/2 cucumber, peeled and chopped</u>

    - <u>1 teaspoon of maple syrup (Dr. Sebi-approved sweetener)</u>

    - <u>1 cup of filtered water</u>

- <u>Portion Measurements: 1 serving (approx. 16 oz.)</u>

- <u>Nutritional Information (per serving):</u>

    - <u>Calories: 50</u>

    - <u>Carbohydrates: 14g</u>

    - <u>Fiber: 2g</u>

    - <u>Protein: 1g</u>

    - <u>Fat: 0g</u>

- <u>Prep Time: 5 minutes</u>

- <u>Instructions:</u>

1. <u>Blend lemon juice, chopped cucumber, maple syrup, and filtered water in a blender.</u>

2. <u>Blend until cleansing and refreshing.</u>

3. <u>Serve in a glass and cleanse your kidneys with a lemonade twist!</u>

<u>**7. Pineapple Papaya Kidney Reviver**</u>

- <u>Ingredients:</u>
    - <u>1 cup of fresh pineapple chunks</u>
    - <u>1/2 cup of fresh papaya chunks</u>
    - <u>1/2 lemon, juiced</u>
    - <u>1 tablespoon of chia seeds</u>
    - <u>1 cup of coconut water</u>
- <u>Portion Measurements: 1 serving (approx. 16 oz.)</u>
- <u>Nutritional Information (per serving):</u>
    - <u>Calories: 190</u>
    - <u>Carbohydrates: 42g</u>
    - <u>Fiber: 7g</u>
    - <u>Protein: 5g</u>
    - <u>Fat: 3g</u>
- <u>Prep Time: 5 minutes</u>
- <u>Instructions:</u>

1. <u>Blend fresh pineapple chunks, papaya chunks, lemon juice, chia seeds, and coconut water in a blender.</u>
2. <u>Blend until reviving and kidney-friendly.</u>
3. <u>Serve in a glass and revive your kidneys with this tropical delight!</u>

<u>**8. Green Kidney Cleanse Supreme**</u>

- <u>Ingredients:</u>

    - <u>2 cups of spinach</u>

    - <u>1/2 cucumber, peeled and chopped</u>

    - <u>1/2 avocado</u>

    - <u>1/2 lime, juiced</u>

    - <u>1 teaspoon of spirulina powder</u>

    - <u>1 teaspoon of chlorella powder</u>

    - <u>1 cup of filtered water</u>

- <u>Portion Measurements: 1 serving (approx. 16 oz.)</u>

- <u>Nutritional Information (per serving):</u>

    - <u>Calories: 170</u>

    - <u>Carbohydrates: 12g</u>

    - <u>Fiber: 5g</u>

    - <u>Protein: 7g</u>

    - <u>Fat: 13g</u>

- <u>Prep Time: 5 minutes</u>

- <u>Instructions:</u>

1. <u>Combine spinach, cucumber, avocado, lime juice, spirulina powder, chlorella powder, and filtered water in a blender.</u>

2. <u>Blend until supremely cleansing and green.</u>

3. <u>Serve in a glass and cleanse your kidneys with the green supreme!</u>

9. Watermelon Kiwi Kidney Cooler

- Ingredients:

    - 1 cup of fresh watermelon chunks

    - 1 kiwi, peeled and chopped

    - 1/2 lemon, juiced

    - 1 teaspoon of flaxseed meal

    - 1 cup of coconut water

- Portion Measurements: 1 serving (approx. 16 oz.)

- Nutritional Information (per serving):

    - Calories: 140

    - Carbohydrates: 34g

    - Fiber: 7g

    - Protein: 3g

    - Fat: 2g

- Prep Time: 5 minutes

- Instructions:

1. Blend watermelon chunks, chopped kiwi, lemon juice, flaxseed meal, and coconut water in a blender.

2. Blend until kidney-cooling and kiwi-delicious.

3. Serve in a glass and chill with the kidney cooler!

<u>**10. Almond Joy Kidney Booster**</u>

- <u>Ingredients:</u>

    - <u>1 cup of unsweetened almond milk</u>

    - <u>1/2 cup of fresh coconut meat</u>

    - <u>1/2 banana</u>

    - <u>1 tablespoon of raw cacao powder</u>

    - <u>1 teaspoon of Dr. Sebi-approved sweetener (e.g., agave nectar)</u>

    - <u>1/2 lime, juiced</u>

- <u>Portion Measurements: 1 serving (approx. 16 oz.)</u>

- <u>Nutritional Information (per serving):</u>

    - <u>Calories: 180</u>

    - <u>Carbohydrates: 20g</u>

    - <u>Fiber: 6g</u>

    - <u>Protein: 4g</u>

    - <u>Fat: 12g</u>

- <u>Prep Time: 5 minutes</u>

- <u>Instructions:</u>

1. <u>Blend unsweetened almond milk, fresh coconut meat, banana, raw cacao powder, sweetener, and lime juice in a blender.</u>

2. <u>Blend until your kidneys get a joyful boost!</u>

3. <u>Serve in a glass and boost your kidneys with almond joy.</u>

Smoothie Benefits

1. Kidney Stone Crusher

- Benefits: Watermelon is rich in water and potassium, which can help flush out toxins and prevent kidney stone formation. Cucumber adds hydration, and mint may soothe inflammation.

2. Gout Buster Blueberry Blast

- Benefits: Blueberries are packed with antioxidants and have anti-inflammatory properties, potentially reducing gout flare-ups. Kale provides essential vitamins.

3. Stone Soothing Spinach Delight

- Benefits: Spinach is a low-purine green leafy vegetable, suitable for gout sufferers. Pineapple offers bromelain, which may aid digestion and reduce inflammation.

4. Cherry Kidney Cleanse

- Benefits: Cherries are known to help lower uric acid levels, reducing the risk of gout attacks. Cucumber provides hydration for kidney health.

5. Turmeric Twist Anti-Inflammatory Smoothie

- Benefits: Turmeric and ginger are powerful anti-inflammatory ingredients, potentially beneficial for both kidney health and gout management.

6. Lemonade Kidney Cleanser

- Benefits: Lemon juice is known for its potential to increase citrate levels in urine, which can help prevent kidney stone formation. Cucumber adds hydration.

7. Pineapple Papaya Kidney Reviver

- Benefits: Pineapple contains bromelain, an enzyme that may aid digestion and reduce inflammation. Papaya is low in purines and may benefit gout sufferers.

8. Green Kidney Cleanse Supreme

- Benefits: Green leafy vegetables like spinach are excellent for kidney health. Spirulina and chlorella offer detoxifying properties.

9. Watermelon Kiwi Kidney Cooler

- Benefits: Watermelon is hydrating and low in purines, making it kidney-friendly. Kiwi adds vitamin C, which may reduce uric acid levels.

10. Almond Joy Kidney Booster

- Benefits: Almonds provide healthy fats and protein, while coconut meat offers hydration. Raw cacao is rich in antioxidants and may reduce inflammation.

These smoothies are designed to include ingredients that can be beneficial for people with kidney stones and gout. However, it's essential to consult with a healthcare professional or a registered dietitian before making significant dietary changes, especially if you have specific medical conditions or concerns.

<u>**Breakfast Recipes**</u>

1. Coconut and Berry Chia Pudding

- Ingredients:
    - 1/4 cup of chia seeds
    - 1 cup of coconut milk (unsweetened)
    - 1 tablespoon of agave nectar (or sweetener of choice)
    - 1/2 cup of mixed berries (e.g., strawberries, blueberries, raspberries)
    - 1 tablespoon of shredded coconut (for garnish)
- Servings: 2
- Portion Measurements: 1 serving (approx. 1/2 cup)
- Nutritional Information (per serving):
    - Calories: 180
    - Carbohydrates: 18g
    - Fiber: 8g
    - Protein: 4g
    - Fat: 11g
- Prep Time: 5 minutes
- Total Time: 5 minutes (plus chilling time)
- Instructions:

1. In a bowl, combine chia seeds and coconut milk.
2. Stir well and let it sit for a few minutes.
3. Add agave nectar and mix thoroughly.
4. Cover and refrigerate for at least 2 hours or overnight until it thickens.
5. Before serving, top with mixed berries and shredded coconut.

2. Alkaline Veggie Omelet

- Ingredients:

    - 4 large organic eggs

    - 1/4 cup of diced bell peppers

    - 1/4 cup of diced onions

    - 1/4 cup of sliced mushrooms

    - 1/4 cup of spinach leaves

    - A pinch of sea salt and black pepper

    - Fresh parsley for garnish (optional)

- Servings: 2

- Portion Measurements (per serving):

    - Calories: 160

    - Carbohydrates: 4g

    - Fiber: 1g

    - Protein: 12g

    - Fat: 10g

- Prep Time: 10 minutes

- Cook Time: 10 minutes

- Total Time: 20 minutes

- Instructions:

1. In a bowl, whisk the eggs until well beaten.

2. Heat a non-stick skillet over medium heat and add diced bell peppers, onions, and sliced mushrooms.

3. Sauté until the vegetables are tender.

4. Add spinach leaves and cook until wilted.

5. Pour the beaten eggs over the vegetables, season with sea salt and black pepper, and cook until the edges start to set.

6. Gently fold the omelet in half and cook for another minute until fully set.

7. Garnish with fresh parsley if desired and serve as a wholesome and alkaline veggie omelet.

<u>**3. Buckwheat Pancakes**</u>

- Ingredients:
    - 1 cup of buckwheat flour
    - 1 cup of almond milk
    - 1 tablespoon of ground flaxseeds
    - 1 teaspoon of vanilla extract
    - Fresh fruit topping (e.g., berries)
- Servings: 2
- Portion Measurements: 1 serving (2 pancakes)
- Nutritional Information (per serving):
    - Calories: 250
    - Carbohydrates: 51g
    - Fiber: 8g
    - Protein: 8g
    - Fat: 3g
- Prep Time: 10 minutes
- Cook Time: 15 minutes
- Total Time: 25 minutes
- Instructions:

1. In a bowl, mix buckwheat flour, almond milk, ground flaxseeds, and vanilla extract until smooth.

2. Heat a non-stick pan over medium heat and lightly grease it.

3. Pour batter onto the pan to make pancakes.

4. Cook for 2-3 minutes on each side until golden brown.

5. Serve with fresh fruit topping.

<u>**4. Avocado and Tomato Toast**</u>

- Ingredients:
  - 2 slices of whole-grain bread (gluten-free if preferred)
  - 1 ripe avocado, mashed
  - 1 tomato, sliced
  - Sea salt and black pepper to taste
- Servings: 2
- Portion Measurements: 1 serving (1 toast)
- Nutritional Information (per serving):
  - Calories: 180
  - Carbohydrates: 22g
  - Fiber: 6g
  - Protein: 4g
  - Fat: 9g
- Prep Time: 5 minutes
- Total Time: 5 minutes
- Instructions:

1. Toast the slices of whole-grain bread.
2. Spread mashed avocado evenly on each slice.
3. Top with tomato slices and season with sea salt and black pepper.
4. Serve immediately.

<u>**5. Plant-Based Oatmeal**</u>

- Ingredients:
    - 1 cup of rolled oats (gluten-free if preferred)
    - 2 cups of almond milk
    - 2 tablespoons of chia seeds
    - Fresh berries (e.g., strawberries, blueberries)
    - 1 tablespoon of maple syrup (or sweetener of choice)
- Servings: 2
- Portion Measurements: 1 serving (approx. 1 cup)
- Nutritional Information (per serving):
    - Calories: 250
    - Carbohydrates: 44g
    - Fiber: 9g
    - Protein: 7g
    - Fat: 5g
- Prep Time: 5 minutes
- Cook Time: 10 minutes
- Total Time: 15 minutes
- Instructions:

1. In a saucepan, combine rolled oats and almond milk.
2. Cook over medium heat, stirring occasionally, until oats are tender (about 10 minutes).
3. Stir in chia seeds and maple syrup.
4. Serve hot, topped with fresh berries.

<u>**6. Alkaline Breakfast Quinoa Bowl**</u>

- Ingredients:
    - 1 cup of cooked quinoa
    - 1/2 cup of almond milk
    - 1/4 cup of chopped nuts (e.g., almonds, walnuts)
    - 1/4 cup of fresh berries (e.g., blueberries, raspberries)
    - 1 tablespoon of agave nectar (or sweetener of choice)
    - A pinch of cinnamon (optional)
- Servings: 2
- Portion Measurements: 1 serving (approx. 1 cup)
- Nutritional Information (per serving):
    - Calories: 250
    - Carbohydrates: 35g
    - Fiber: 6g
    - Protein: 7g
    - Fat: 10g
- Prep Time: 5 minutes
- Total Time: 5 minutes
- Instructions:

1. In a bowl, combine cooked quinoa and almond milk.

2. Top with chopped nuts, fresh berries, agave nectar, and a pinch of cinnamon.

3. Stir well and serve.

<u>**7. Dr. Sebi's Plantain Pancakes**</u>

- Ingredients:
    - 2 ripe plantains
    - 1/4 cup of almond milk
    - 1 teaspoon of vanilla extract
    - A pinch of sea salt
    - Coconut oil for cooking
- Servings: 2
- Portion Measurements: 1 serving (2-3 pancakes)
- Nutritional Information (per serving):
    - Calories: 180
    - Carbohydrates: 43g
    - Fiber: 3g
    - Protein: 2g
    - Fat: 1g
- Prep Time: 10 minutes
- Cook Time: 10 minutes
- Total Time: 20 minutes
- Instructions:

1. Peel and chop the ripe plantains.

2. In a blender, combine the plantains, almond milk, vanilla extract, and a pinch of sea salt. Blend until smooth.

3. Heat a non-stick skillet or griddle over medium heat and lightly grease with coconut oil.

4. Pour small amounts of the plantain batter onto the skillet to make pancakes.

5. Cook for 2-3 minutes on each side until golden brown.

6. Serve with fresh fruit or a drizzle of agave nectar.

<u>**8. Alkaline Tofu Scramble**</u>

- Ingredients:
    - 1/2 block of organic tofu, crumbled
    - 1/4 cup of diced bell peppers
    - 1/4 cup of diced onions
    - 1/4 cup of chopped tomatoes
    - 1/2 teaspoon of turmeric powder
    - A pinch of sea salt and black pepper
    - Fresh cilantro for garnish (optional)
- Servings: 2
- Portion Measurements (per serving):
    - Calories: 110
    - Carbohydrates: 6g
    - Fiber: 2g
    - Protein: 9g
    - Fat: 6g
- Prep Time: 10 minutes
- Cook Time: 10 minutes
- Total Time: 20 minutes
- Instructions:

1. In a pan, sauté diced bell peppers and onions until they become tender.

2. Add crumbled tofu, chopped tomatoes, turmeric powder, sea salt, and black pepper.

3. Cook and stir until the tofu is heated through and coated with the spices.

4. Garnish with fresh cilantro if desired and serve as an alkaline tofu scramble.

<u>**9. Mango and Coconut Parfait**</u>

- Ingredients:

    - 1 ripe mango, diced

    - 1 cup of coconut yogurt (or coconut milk yogurt)

    - 2 tablespoons of shredded coconut

    - 1 tablespoon of agave nectar (or sweetener of choice)

- Servings: 2

- Portion Measurements: 1 serving (approx. 1 cup)

- Nutritional Information (per serving):

    - Calories: 180

    - Carbohydrates: 35g

    - Fiber: 4g

    - Protein: 2g

    - Fat: 5g

- Prep Time: 10 minutes

- Total Time: 10 minutes

- Instructions:

1. In serving glasses, layer diced mango, coconut yogurt, and shredded coconut.

2. Drizzle agave nectar on top.

3. Repeat the layers as desired.

4. Serve chilled.

<u>**10. Dr. Sebi's Almond Butter Toast**</u>

- Ingredients:
    - 2 slices of whole-grain bread (gluten-free if preferred)
    - 2 tablespoons of almond butter
    - Sliced banana for topping
    - A sprinkle of cinnamon (optional)
- Servings: 2
- Portion Measurements: 1 serving (1 toast)
- Nutritional Information (per serving):
    - Calories: 220
    - Carbohydrates: 30g
    - Fiber: 5g
    - Protein: 7g
    - Fat: 9g
- Prep Time: 5 minutes
- Total Time: 5 minutes
- Instructions:

1. Toast the slices of whole-grain bread.

2. Spread almond butter evenly on each slice.

3. Top with sliced banana and a sprinkle of cinnamon if desired.

4. Serve immediately.

<u>Lunch Recipes</u>

1. Chickpea and Vegetable Salad

- Ingredients:
    - 1 can of chickpeas (15 ounces), drained and rinsed
    - 1 cup of cherry tomatoes, halved
    - 1 cucumber, diced
    - 1/2 red onion, finely chopped
    - 1/4 cup of fresh parsley, chopped
    - 2 tablespoons of olive oil
    - 1 lemon (juiced)
    - Salt and pepper to taste
- Servings: 2
- Portion Measurements: 1 serving (approx. 2 cups)
- Nutritional Information (per serving):
    - Calories: 280
    - Carbohydrates: 36g
    - Fiber: 10g
    - Protein: 10g
    - Fat: 12g
- Prep Time: 15 minutes
- Total Time: 15 minutes
- Instructions:

1. In a large bowl, combine the chickpeas, cherry tomatoes, cucumber, red onion, and fresh parsley.

2. In a separate small bowl, whisk together the olive oil, lemon juice, salt, and pepper.

3. Drizzle the dressing over the salad and toss to combine.

4. Serve immediately or refrigerate until ready to eat.

<u>**2. Alkaline Baked Cod with Tomatoes**</u>

- Ingredients:
    - 4 cod fillets
    - 2 cups of diced tomatoes
    - 1/4 cup of chopped fresh basil
    - 2 tablespoons of olive oil
    - 2 cloves of garlic, minced
    - Salt and pepper to taste
- Servings: 4
- Portion Measurements: 1 serving (1 cod fillet with tomato topping)
- Nutritional Information (per serving):
    - Calories: 180
    - Carbohydrates: 5g
    - Fiber: 1g
    - Protein: 25g
    - Fat: 7g
- Prep Time: 10 minutes
- Cook Time: 20 minutes
- Total Time: 30 minutes
- Instructions:
1. Preheat your oven to 375°F (190°C).
2. In a bowl, mix diced tomatoes, chopped fresh basil, olive oil, minced garlic, salt, and pepper.
3. Place cod fillets in a baking dish and top each with the tomato mixture.
4. Bake for 15-20 minutes or until the cod flakes easily with a fork.
5. Serve hot.

<u>**3. Lentil and Vegetable Soup**</u>

- Ingredients:
    - 1 cup of green or brown lentils, rinsed
    - 4 cups of vegetable broth
    - 1 onion, chopped
    - 2 carrots, diced
    - 2 celery stalks, diced
    - 2 cloves of garlic, minced
    - 1 teaspoon of ground cumin
    - 1 teaspoon of ground coriander
    - 1/2 teaspoon of turmeric
    - Salt and pepper to taste
    - Fresh lemon juice for serving
- Servings: 4
- Portion Measurements: 1 serving (approx. 1.5 cups)
- Nutritional Information (per serving):
    - Calories: 220
    - Carbohydrates: 39g
    - Fiber: 13g
    - Protein: 14g
    - Fat: 1g
- Prep Time: 10 minutes
- Cook Time: 30 minutes
- Total Time: 40 minutes
- Instructions:

1. In a large pot, heat a bit of vegetable broth over medium heat.

2. Add chopped onion, carrots, celery, and garlic. Cook until softened, about 5 minutes.

3. Stir in cumin, coriander, and turmeric. Cook for another 2 minutes.

4. Add lentils and the remaining vegetable broth. Bring to a boil, then reduce heat to simmer. Cover and cook for 20-25 minutes or until lentils are tender.

5. Season with salt and pepper.

6. Serve hot with a squeeze of fresh lemon juice.

4. Chickpea Curry

- Ingredients:
    - 1 can of chickpeas (15 ounces), drained and rinsed
    - 1 onion, chopped
    - 2 cloves of garlic, minced
    - 1 can of diced tomatoes (14 ounces)
    - 1 can of coconut milk (14 ounces)
    - 2 tablespoons of curry powder
    - 1 teaspoon of ground cumin
    - 1/2 teaspoon of ground coriander
    - Salt and pepper to taste
    - Fresh cilantro for garnish
- Servings: 4
- Portion Measurements: 1 serving (approx. 1 cup)
- Nutritional Information (per serving):
    - Calories: 320
    - Carbohydrates: 30g
    - Fiber: 8g
    - Protein: 8g
    - Fat: 20g
- Prep Time: 10 minutes
- Cook Time: 20 minutes
- Total Time: 30 minutes
- Instructions:

1. In a large skillet, heat a bit of water or vegetable broth over medium heat.
2. Add chopped onion and minced garlic. Cook until onion is translucent, about 3 minutes.
3. Stir in curry powder, ground cumin, and ground coriander. Cook for another 2 minutes.
4. Add chickpeas, diced tomatoes, and coconut milk. Bring to a simmer.
5. Cook for 15 minutes, stirring occasionally.
6. Season with salt and pepper.
7. Serve hot, garnished with fresh cilantro.

<u>**5. Alkaline Veggie Wrap**</u>

- Ingredients:
    - Collard greens leaves (as the wrap)
    - Hummus (store-bought or homemade)
    - Avocado, sliced
    - Bell peppers, thinly sliced
    - Cucumber, thinly sliced
    - Carrots, grated
    - Sprouts (e.g., alfalfa or broccoli sprouts)
- Servings: 2
- Portion Measurements: 1 serving (1 wrap)
- Nutritional Information (per serving):
    - Calories: 150
    - Carbohydrates: 15g
    - Fiber: 7g
    - Protein: 4g
    - Fat: 9g
- Prep Time: 15 minutes
- Total Time: 15 minutes
- Instructions:

1. Wash and trim the stem of collard greens leaves to make them suitable for wrapping.
2. Lay a collard green leaf flat and spread a generous amount of hummus over it.
3. Layer with avocado slices, bell peppers, cucumber, grated carrots, and sprouts.
4. Fold the sides of the leaf inwards and then roll it up like a burrito.
5. Repeat with remaining leaves and fillings.
6. Serve immediately.

<u>**6. Alkaline Quinoa Salad**</u>

- Ingredients:
    - 1 cup of cooked quinoa
    - 1/2 cup of diced red bell pepper
    - 1/2 cup of diced yellow bell pepper
    - 1/2 cup of diced cucumber
    - 1/4 cup of chopped fresh parsley
    - 1/4 cup of chopped fresh cilantro
    - Juice of 1 lemon
    - 2 tablespoons of olive oil
    - Salt and pepper to taste
- Servings: 2
- Portion Measurements: 1 serving (approx. 1.5 cups)
- Nutritional Information (per serving):
    - Calories: 250
    - Carbohydrates: 29g
    - Fiber: 5g
    - Protein: 4g
    - Fat: 14g
- Prep Time: 15 minutes
- Total Time: 15 minutes
- Instructions:

1. In a large bowl, combine cooked quinoa, diced red bell pepper, diced yellow bell pepper, diced cucumber, fresh parsley, and fresh cilantro.

2. In a separate small bowl, whisk together lemon juice, olive oil, salt, and pepper.

3. Drizzle the dressing over the salad and toss to combine.

4. Serve chilled.

<u>**7. Alkaline Stuffed Bell Peppers**</u>

- Ingredients:

    - 4 large bell peppers (red, yellow, or green)

    - 1 cup of cooked quinoa

    - 1 can of black beans (15 ounces), drained and rinsed

    - 1 cup of corn kernels (fresh or frozen)

    - 1/2 cup of diced tomatoes

    - 1/2 teaspoon of chili powder

    - 1/2 teaspoon of ground cumin

    - Salt and pepper to taste

    - Fresh cilantro for garnish

- Servings: 4

- Portion Measurements: 1 serving (1 stuffed bell pepper)

- Nutritional Information (per serving):

    - Calories: 250

    - Carbohydrates: 48g

    - Fiber: 12g

    - Protein: 12g

    - Fat: 2g

- Prep Time: 20 minutes

- Cook Time: 30 minutes

- Total Time: 50 minutes

- Instructions:

1. Preheat the oven to 375°F (190°C).

2. Cut the tops off the bell peppers and remove the seeds and membranes.

3. In a large bowl, combine cooked quinoa, black beans, corn kernels, diced tomatoes, chili powder, ground cumin, salt, and pepper.

4. Stuff each bell pepper with the quinoa mixture.

5. Place the stuffed bell peppers in a baking dish.

6. Cover with foil and bake for 30-35 minutes or until the peppers are tender.

7. Garnish with fresh cilantro before serving.

<u>**8. Alkaline Spinach and Mushroom Salad**</u>

- Ingredients:

    - 4 cups of fresh spinach leaves

    - 1 cup of sliced mushrooms

    - 1/4 cup of diced red onion

    - 1/4 cup of sliced almonds

    - Juice of 1 lemon

    - 2 tablespoons of olive oil

    - Salt and pepper to taste

- Servings: 2

- Portion Measurements: 1 serving (approx. 2 cups)

- Nutritional Information (per serving):

    - Calories: 180

    - Carbohydrates: 9g

    - Fiber: 3g

    - Protein: 4g

    - Fat: 14g

- Prep Time: 10 minutes

- Total Time: 10 minutes

- Instructions:

1.   In a large bowl, combine fresh spinach leaves, sliced mushrooms, diced red onion, and sliced almonds.

2.   In a separate small bowl, whisk together lemon juice, olive oil, salt, and pepper.

3.   Drizzle the dressing over the salad and toss to combine.

4.   Serve immediately.

<u>**9. Alkaline Zucchini Noodles with Pesto**</u>

- Ingredients:

    - 2 large zucchinis, spiral-ized into noodles

    - 1 cup of fresh basil leaves

    - 1/4 cup of pine nuts

    - 2 cloves of garlic

    - Juice of 1 lemon

    - 2 tablespoons of nutritional yeast

    - 2 tablespoons of olive oil

    - Salt and pepper to taste

    - Cherry tomatoes for garnish

- Servings: 2

- Portion Measurements: 1 serving (approx. 1.5 cups)

- Nutritional Information (per serving):

    - Calories: 200

    - Carbohydrates: 10g

    - Fiber: 4g

    - Protein: 5g

    - Fat: 16g

- Prep Time: 15 minutes

- Total Time: 15 minutes

- Instructions:

1. In a food processor, combine fresh basil leaves, pine nuts, garlic, lemon juice, nutritional yeast, olive oil, salt, and pepper. Blend until smooth to make the pesto sauce.

2. In a large bowl, toss the spiral-ized zucchini noodles with the pesto sauce until well coated.

3. Garnish with cherry tomatoes before serving.

10. Alkaline Coconut Lime Mahi-Mahi

- Ingredients:
    - 4 mahi-mahi fillets
    - 1 can of coconut milk (13.5 ounces)
    - Juice and zest of 2 limes
    - 2 cloves of garlic, minced
    - 1 teaspoon of ground turmeric
    - 1/2 teaspoon of ground cumin
    - Salt and pepper to taste
    - Chopped fresh cilantro for garnish
- Servings: 4
- Portion Measurements: 1 serving (1 mahi-mahi fillet with sauce)
- Nutritional Information (per serving):
    - Calories: 280
    - Carbohydrates: 3g
    - Fiber: 1g
    - Protein: 30g
    - Fat: 16g
- Prep Time: 10 minutes
- Cook Time: 15 minutes
- Total Time: 25 minutes
- Instructions:

1. In a saucepan, combine coconut milk, lime juice, lime zest, minced garlic, ground turmeric, ground cumin, salt, and pepper.

2. Heat the mixture over medium heat until it begins to simmer. Reduce heat and let it simmer for 5 minutes.

3. Season mahi-mahi fillets with salt and pepper and grill them for about 4-5 minutes per side until cooked through.

4. Serve mahi-mahi fillets with the coconut lime sauce and garnish with chopped fresh cilantro.

<u>**Dinner Recipes**</u>

1. Alkaline Grilled Salmon

- Ingredients:
    - 4 salmon fillets
    - 1/4 cup of chopped fresh parsley
    - 2 tablespoons of olive oil
    - 1 lemon, sliced
    - 2 cloves of garlic, minced
    - Salt and pepper to taste
- Servings: 4
- Portion Measurements: 1 serving (1 salmon fillet)
- Nutritional Information (per serving):
    - Calories: 300
    - Carbohydrates: 2g
    - Fiber: 1g
    - Protein: 25g
    - Fat: 20g
- Prep Time: 10 minutes
- Cook Time: 15 minutes
- Total Time: 25 minutes
- Instructions:

1. Preheat your grill to medium-high heat.
2. In a bowl, mix chopped parsley, olive oil, minced garlic, salt, and pepper.
3. Brush the mixture over both sides of the salmon fillets.
4. Place salmon fillets on the grill and cook for about 6-8 minutes per side, or until the salmon flakes easily with a fork.
5. Serve with lemon slices.

<u>**2. Alkaline Veggie Stir-Fry**</u>

- Ingredients:
    - 2 cups of broccoli florets
    - 1 cup of sliced bell peppers (red, yellow, and green)
    - 1 cup of sliced mushrooms
    - 1 cup of sliced zucchini
    - 1 cup of sliced yellow squash
    - 1/2 cup of sliced red onion
    - 2 cloves of garlic, minced
    - 2 tablespoons of coconut oil
    - 2 tablespoons of low-sodium soy sauce (or tamari for a gluten-free option)
    - 1 teaspoon of grated ginger
    - 1/2 teaspoon of ground turmeric
    - Salt and pepper to taste
- Servings: 4
- Portion Measurements: 1 serving (approx. 2 cups)
- Nutritional Information (per serving):
    - Calories: 150
    - Carbohydrates: 15g
    - Fiber: 4g
    - Protein: 4g
    - Fat: 9g
- Prep Time: 15 minutes
- Cook Time: 15 minutes
- Total Time: 30 minutes
- Instructions:

1. In a large skillet, heat coconut oil over medium-high heat.

2. Add minced garlic and grated ginger. Sauté for about 1 minute until fragrant.

3. Add broccoli florets, bell peppers, mushrooms, zucchini, yellow squash, and red onion to the skillet. Stir-fry for 5-7 minutes until the vegetables are tender-crisp.

4. In a small bowl, whisk together low-sodium soy sauce and ground turmeric.

5. Pour the sauce over the stir-fried vegetables and toss to combine.

6. Season with salt and pepper.

7. Serve hot.

3. Alkaline Baked Portobello Mushrooms

- Ingredients:
    - 4 large Portobello mushrooms, stems removed
    - 1 cup of diced tomatoes
    - 1/2 cup of diced bell peppers
    - 1/2 cup of diced onions
    - 2 cloves of garlic, minced
    - 2 tablespoons of olive oil
    - 1 teaspoon of oregano
    - A pinch of sea salt and black pepper
    - Fresh basil for garnish (optional)
- Servings: 4
- Nutritional Information (per serving):
    - Calories: 90
    - Carbohydrates: 8g
    - Fiber: 3g
    - Protein: 3g
    - Fat: 6g
- Prep Time: 15 minutes
- Cook Time: 20 minutes
- Total Time: 35 minutes
- Instructions:

1. Preheat your oven to 375°F (190°C).
2. In a bowl, mix diced tomatoes, bell peppers, onions, garlic, olive oil, oregano, sea salt, and black pepper.
3. Place Portobello mushrooms on a baking sheet, gill-side up.
4. Stuff each mushroom with the tomato mixture.
5. Bake in the preheated oven for about 20 minutes until mushrooms are tender.
6. Garnish with fresh basil if desired.
7. Serve as a delightful and alkaline dinner option.

<u>**4. Alkaline Spaghetti Squash with Marinara Sauce**</u>

- Ingredients:
    - 1 large spaghetti squash
    - 2 cups of Alkaline tomato sauce (see recipe below)
    - 1/4 cup of nutritional yeast
    - 1/4 cup of fresh basil leaves, chopped
    - Salt and pepper to taste
- Servings: 4
- Portion Measurements: 1 serving (approx. 1 cup)
- Nutritional Information (per serving):
    - Calories: 120
    - Carbohydrates: 30g
    - Fiber: 6g
    - Protein: 4g
    - Fat: 1g
- Prep Time: 10 minutes
- Cook Time: 45 minutes
- Total Time: 55 minutes
- Instructions:

1. Preheat the oven to 375°F (190°C).
2. Cut the spaghetti squash in half lengthwise and scoop out the seeds.
3. Place the squash halves, cut-side down, on a baking sheet.
4. Bake for 45 minutes or until the squash is tender and the flesh easily shreds into spaghetti-like strands with a fork.
5. Use a fork to scrape the squash flesh into a bowl, creating "spaghetti."
6. Heat the Alkaline tomato sauce in a saucepan over low heat.
7. Serve the spaghetti squash topped with marinara sauce, nutritional yeast, fresh basil, salt, and pepper.

<u>**5. Alkaline Lentil and Vegetable Stew**</u>

- Ingredients:
    - 1 cup of dried green lentils, rinsed and drained
    - 4 cups of vegetable broth
    - 1 cup of diced tomatoes
    - 1 cup of diced carrots
    - 1 cup of diced celery
    - 1 cup of diced bell peppers (red, yellow, or green)
    - 1/2 cup of diced onions
    - 2 cloves of garlic, minced
    - 1/2 teaspoon of ground turmeric
    - 1/2 teaspoon of ground cumin
    - 1/2 teaspoon of paprika
    - Salt and pepper to taste
    - Fresh parsley for garnish
- Servings: 4
- Portion Measurements: 1 serving (approx. 1.5 cups)
- Nutritional Information (per serving):
    - Calories: 200
    - Carbohydrates: 36g
    - Fiber: 15g
    - Protein: 13g
    - Fat: 1g
- Prep Time: 15 minutes
- Cook Time: 25 minutes
- Total Time: 40 minutes
- Instructions:

1. In a large pot, combine dried green lentils, vegetable broth, diced tomatoes, diced carrots, diced celery, diced bell peppers, diced onions, minced garlic, ground turmeric, ground cumin, paprika, salt, and pepper.

2. Bring the mixture to a boil, then reduce the heat to low, cover, and simmer for 20-25 minutes or until the lentils and vegetables are tender.

3. Serve hot, garnished with fresh parsley.

<u>**6. Alkaline Herb-Crusted Tilapia**</u>

- Ingredients:
    - 4 tilapia fillets
    - 1/4 cup of chopped fresh parsley
    - 1/4 cup of chopped fresh cilantro
    - 2 tablespoons of almond meal
    - 2 tablespoons of olive oil
    - 1 lemon, sliced
    - Salt and pepper to taste
- Servings: 4
- Portion Measurements: 1 serving (1 tilapia fillet)
- Nutritional Information (per serving):
    - Calories: 200
    - Carbohydrates: 1g
    - Fiber: 0.5g
    - Protein: 25g
    - Fat: 10g
- Prep Time: 10 minutes
- Cook Time: 15 minutes
- Total Time: 25 minutes
- Instructions:

1. Preheat your oven to 375°F (190°C).
2. In a bowl, mix chopped fresh parsley, chopped fresh cilantro, almond meal, olive oil, salt, and pepper.
3. Place tilapia fillets on a baking sheet lined with parchment paper.
4. Spread the herb mixture evenly over the top of each fillet.
5. Bake for 12-15 minutes or until the tilapia is cooked and flakes easily with a fork.
6. Serve with lemon slices.
7. In a small bowl, whisk together low-sodium soy sauce and ground turmeric.
8. Pour the sauce over the stir-fried cauliflower rice and vegetables and toss to combine.
9. Season with salt and pepper.
10. Serve hot.

<u>**7. Alkaline Quinoa and Black Bean Bowl**</u>

- Ingredients:

    - 2 cups of cooked quinoa

    - 1 can of black beans (15 ounces), drained and rinsed

    - 1 cup of diced tomatoes

    - 1 cup of corn kernels (fresh or frozen)

    - 1/2 cup of diced red onion

    - 1/2 cup of diced red bell pepper

    - 1/4 cup of diced avocado

    - Juice of 1 lime

    - 2 tablespoons of olive oil

    - 1/2 teaspoon of ground cumin

    - Salt and pepper to taste

- Servings: 4
- Portion Measurements: 1 serving (approx. 2 cups)
- Nutritional Information (per serving):

    - Calories: 280

    - Carbohydrates: 48g

    - Fiber: 12g

    - Protein: 9g

    - Fat: 7g

- Prep Time: 15 minutes
- Total Time: 15 minutes
- Instructions:

1. In a large bowl, combine cooked quinoa, black beans, diced tomatoes, corn kernels, diced red onion, diced red bell pepper, and diced avocado.

2. In a separate small bowl, whisk together lime juice, olive oil, ground cumin, salt, and pepper.

3. Drizzle the dressing over the bowl and toss to combine.

4. Serve immediately.

<u>**8. Alkaline Lemon Garlic Shrimp**</u>

- Ingredients:
    - 1 pound of large shrimp, peeled and deveined
    - 2 tablespoons of olive oil
    - 4 cloves of garlic, minced
    - Juice of 2 lemons
    - 1 teaspoon of dried oregano
    - Salt and pepper to taste
    - Chopped fresh parsley for garnish
- Servings: 4
- Portion Measurements: 1 serving (1/4 of the recipe)
- Nutritional Information (per serving):
    - Calories: 150
    - Carbohydrates: 4g
    - Fiber: 0.5g
    - Protein: 18g
    - Fat: 8g
- Prep Time: 10 minutes
- Cook Time: 5 minutes
- Total Time: 15 minutes
- Instructions:

1. Heat olive oil in a large skillet over medium-high heat.
2. Add minced garlic and sauté for about 30 seconds until fragrant.
3. Add shrimp to the skillet and cook for 2-3 minutes per side, or until they turn pink and opaque.
4. Pour lemon juice over the shrimp and sprinkle with dried oregano, salt, and pepper.
5. Stir well to combine and cook for another minute.
6. Garnish with chopped fresh parsley before serving.

<u>**9. Alkaline Spinach and Avocado Salad**</u>

- Ingredients:
    - 4 cups of fresh spinach leaves
    - 1 avocado, diced
    - 1/4 cup of sliced almonds
    - Juice of 1 lemon
    - 2 tablespoons of olive oil
    - Salt and pepper to taste
- Servings: 2
- Portion Measurements: 1 serving (approx. 2 cups)
- Nutritional Information (per serving):
    - Calories: 220
    - Carbohydrates: 10g
    - Fiber: 6g
    - Protein: 4g
    - Fat: 18g
- Prep Time: 10 minutes
- Total Time: 10 minutes
- Instructions:

1. In a large bowl, combine fresh spinach leaves, diced avocado, and sliced almonds.

2. In a separate small bowl, whisk together lemon juice, olive oil, salt, and pepper.

3. Drizzle the dressing over the salad and toss to combine.

4. Serve immediately.

<u>**10. Alkaline Quinoa and Vegetable Stir-Fry**</u>

- Ingredients:
    - 2 cups of cooked quinoa
    - 1 cup of sliced mushrooms
    - 1 cup of sliced bell peppers (red, yellow, and green)
    - 1 cup of sliced zucchini
    - 1 cup of sliced yellow squash
    - 1 cup of sliced broccoli florets
    - 1/2 cup of diced onions
    - 2 cloves of garlic, minced
    - 2 tablespoons of coconut oil
    - 2 tablespoons of low-sodium soy sauce (or tamari for a gluten-free option)
    - 1 teaspoon of grated ginger
    - 1/2 teaspoon of ground turmeric
    - Salt and pepper to taste
- Servings: 4
- Portion Measurements: 1 serving (approx. 2 cups)
- Nutritional Information (per serving):
    - Calories: 250
    - Carbohydrates: 38g
    - Fiber: 7g
    - Protein: 8g
    - Fat: 9g
- Prep Time: 15 minutes
- Cook Time: 15 minutes
- Total Time: 30 minutes
- Instructions:

1. In a large skillet, heat coconut oil over medium-high heat.
2. Add minced garlic and grated ginger. Sauté for about 1 minute until fragrant.
3. Add sliced mushrooms, bell peppers, zucchini, yellow squash, broccoli florets, and diced onions to the skillet. Stir-fry for 5-7 minutes until the vegetables are tender-crisp.
4. In a small bowl, whisk together low-sodium soy sauce and ground turmeric.
5. Pour the sauce over the stir-fried quinoa and vegetables and toss to combine.
6. Season with salt and pepper.
7. Serve hot.

<u>7 – Day Meal Plan</u>

(This is just one example of our 7-day meal plan. With 10 breakfast options, 10 lunch choices, and 10 dinner recipes, you can create an astonishing 1 quintillion unique 7-day meal plan combinations.)

<u>Day 1:</u>

Breakfast: Alkaline Veggie Omelet

Lunch: Chickpea and Vegetable Salad

Dinner: Alkaline Grilled Salmon

<u>Day 2:</u>

Breakfast: Buckwheat Pancakes

Lunch: Alkaline Baked Cod with Tomatoes

Dinner: Alkaline Spaghetti Squash with Marinara Sauce

<u>Day 3:</u>

Breakfast: Alkaline Breakfast Quinoa Bowl

Lunch: Alkaline Veggie Wrap

Dinner: Alkaline Spinach and Avocado Salad

<u>Day 4:</u>

Breakfast: Alkaline Tofu Scramble

Lunch: Alkaline Quinoa Salad

Dinner: Alkaline Veggie Stir-Fry

<u>Day 5:</u>

Breakfast: Dr. Sebi's Plantain Pancakes

Lunch: Alkaline Stuffed Bell Peppers

Dinner: Alkaline Lemon Garlic Shrimp

<u>Day 6:</u>

Breakfast: Mango and Coconut Parfait

Lunch: Alkaline Zucchini Noodles with Pesto

Dinner: Alkaline Quinoa and Vegetable Stir-Fry

<u>Day 7:</u>

Breakfast: Avocado and Tomato Toast

Lunch: Alkaline Coconut Lime Mahi-Mahi

Dinner: Alkaline Baked Portobello Mushrooms

****This meal plan provides a variety of balanced and nutritious meals, including a mix of whole grains, lean proteins, healthy fats, and plenty of vegetables and fruits. You can adjust portion sizes to meet your specific dietary needs and preferences.**